I Already Love You

By: Corinne Lamontagne

Balboa Press books may be ordered through booksellers or by contacting:

Balboa Press
A Division of Hay House
1663 Liberty Drive
Bloomington, IN 47403
www.balboapress.com
1 (877) 407-4847

ISBN: 978-1-9822-1097-7 (SC)
978-1-9822-1098-4 (e)

Library of Congress Control Number: 2018910130

Print information available on the last page.

Balboa Press rev. date: 11/13/2018

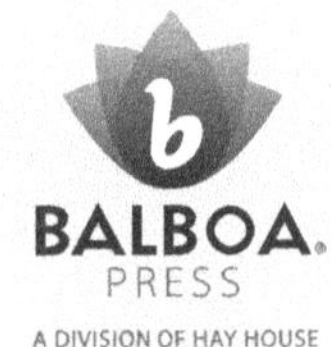

Dedication

To **ALL** God's little miracles. May you always know how much He loves you.

Acknowledgement

Thank you God for using me
to share Your great love.

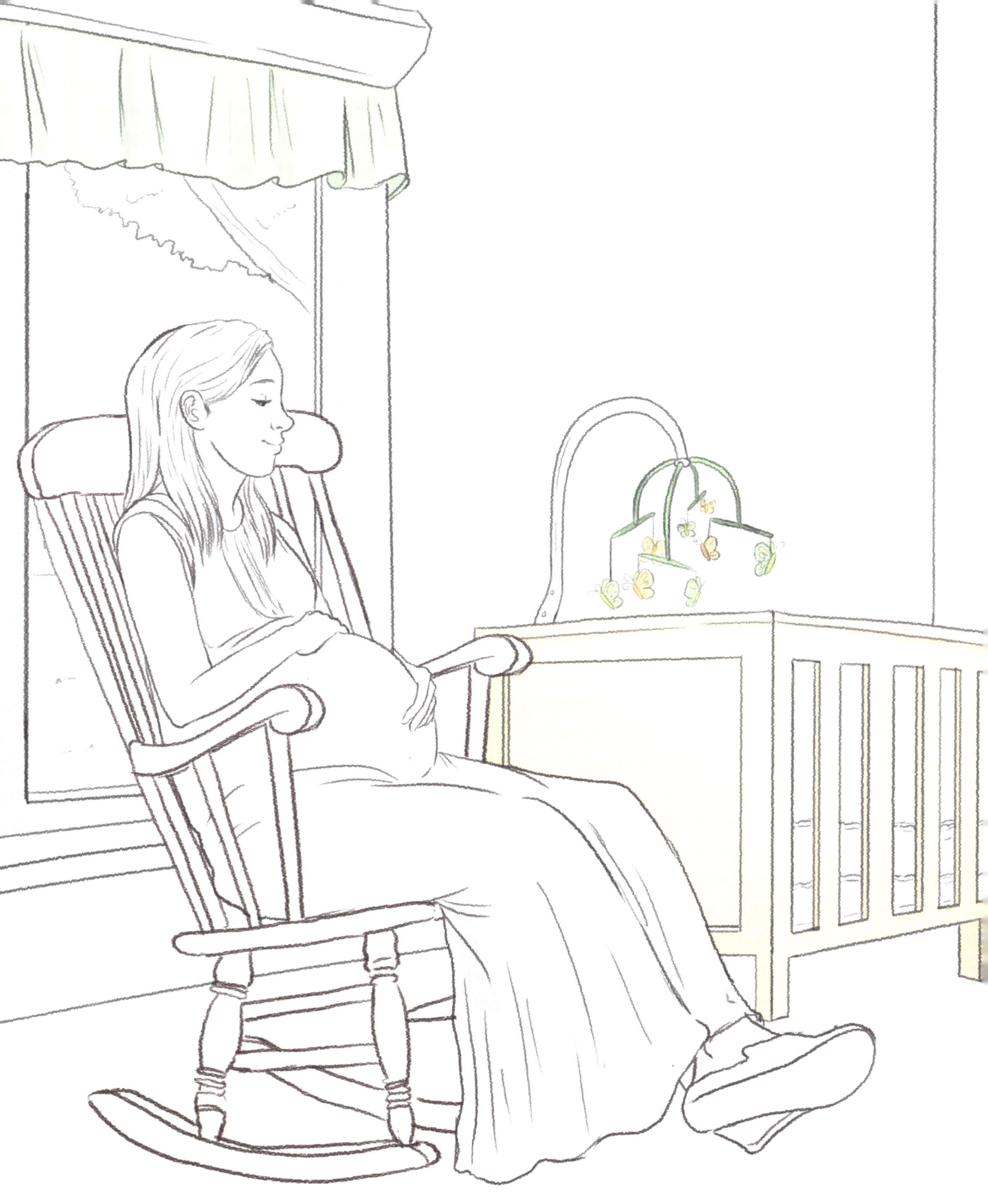

I already love you...my little miracle.

My heart is filled with a love so great,
words can only begin to describe.

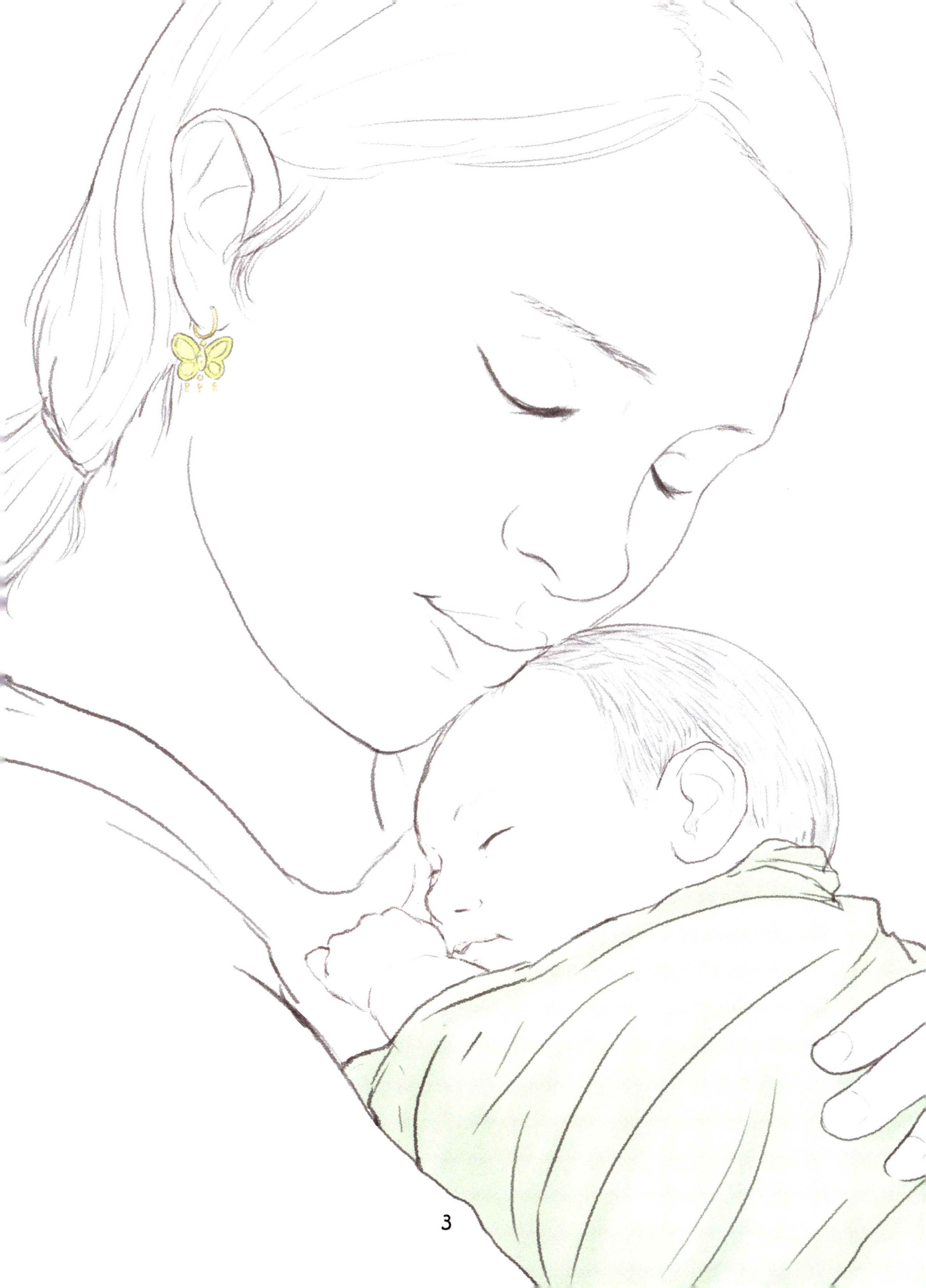

I wonder...

Will you have my eyes, my nose, your daddy's smile?

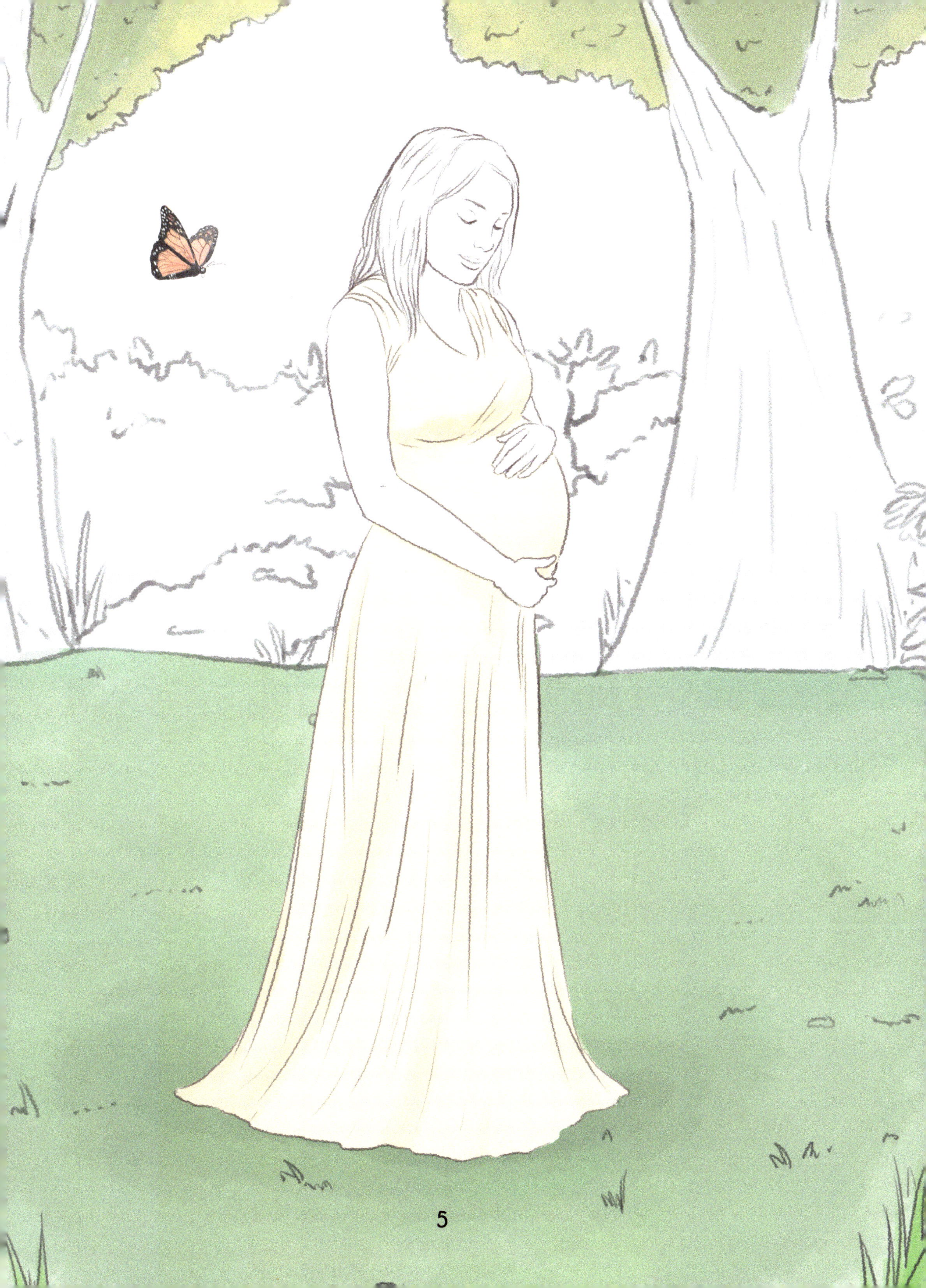

I pray... 

You always know how much you are loved.

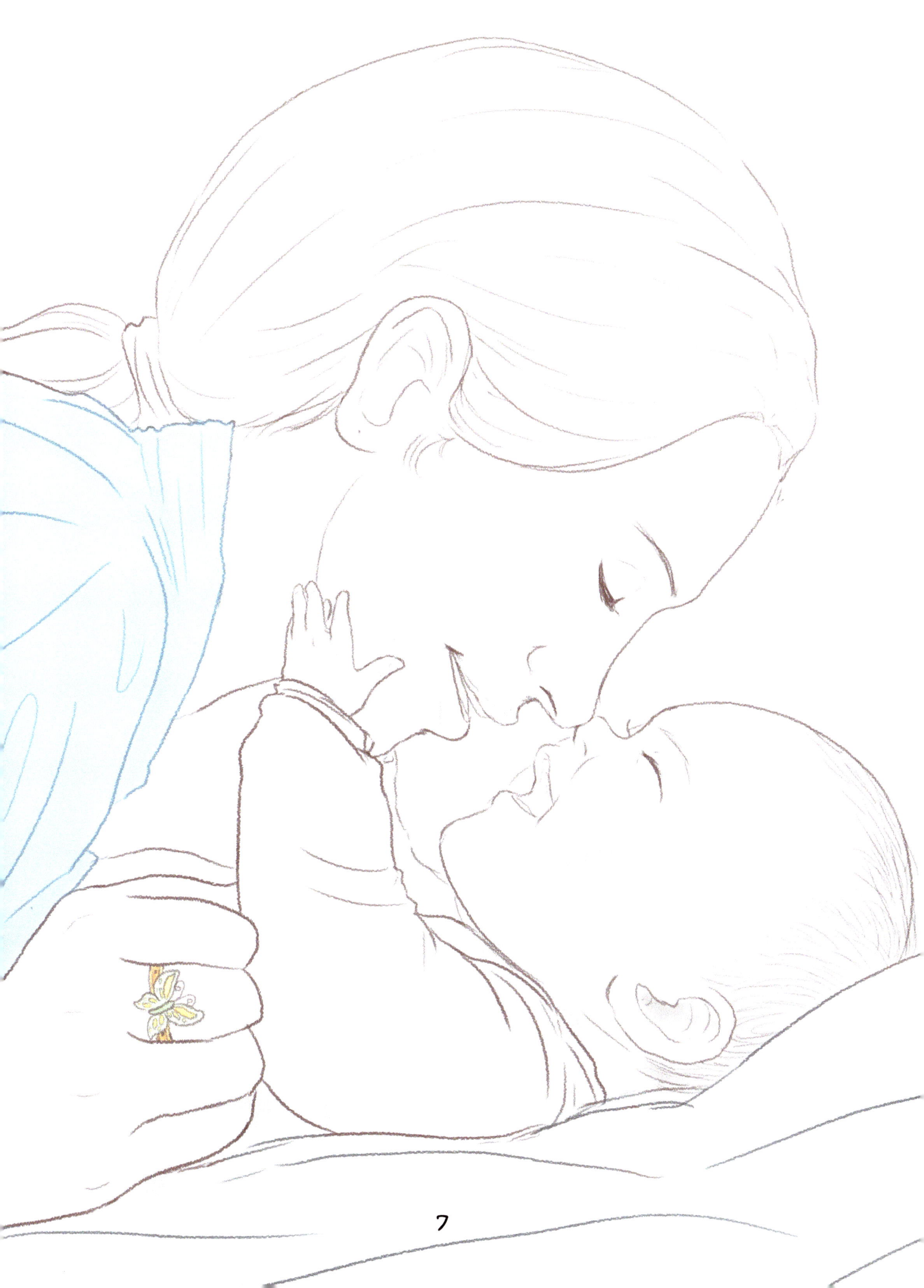

I feel you...

Every flutter, a reminder of God's amazing love.

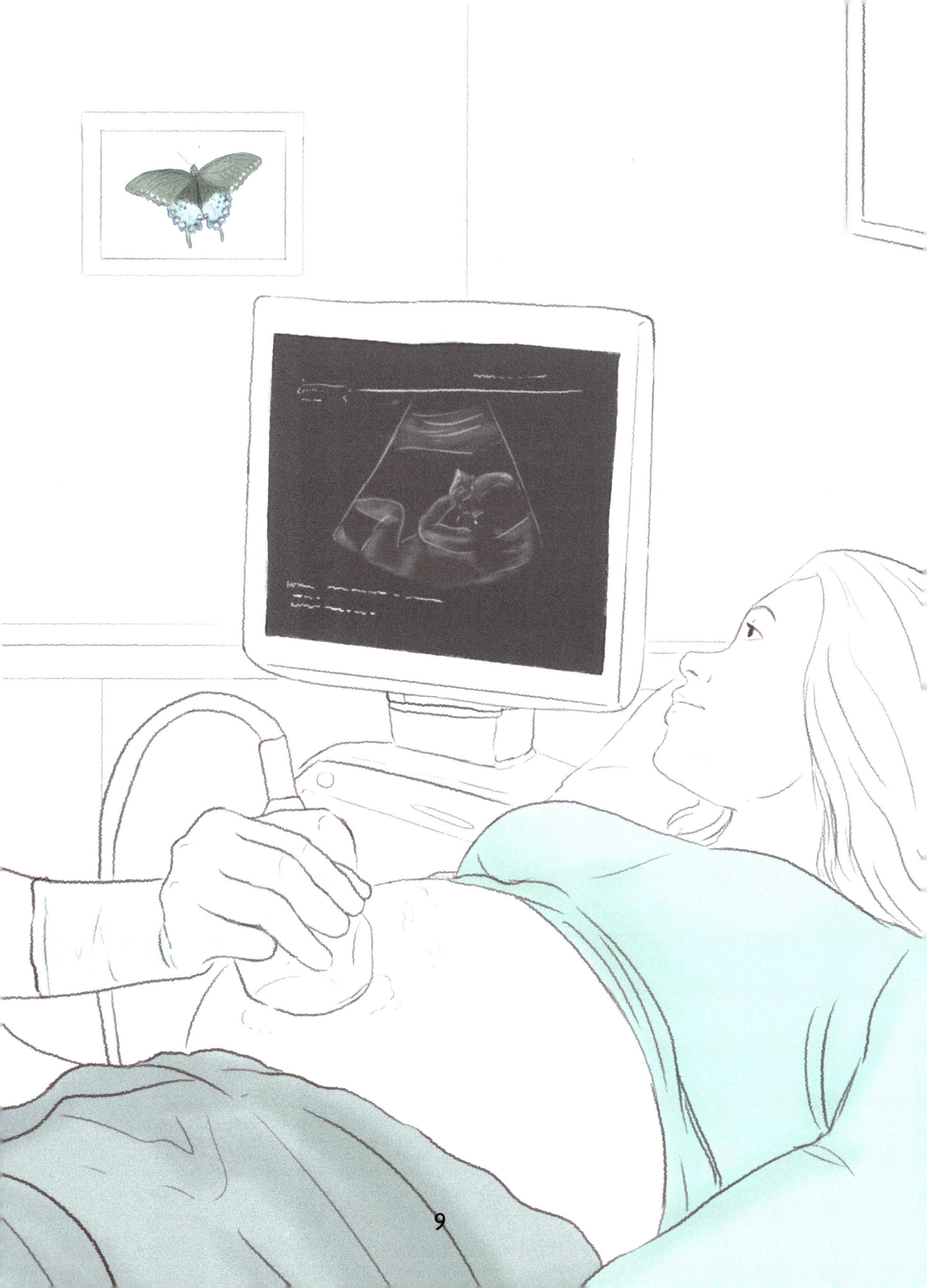

Entrusted to me to love, guide, and protect.

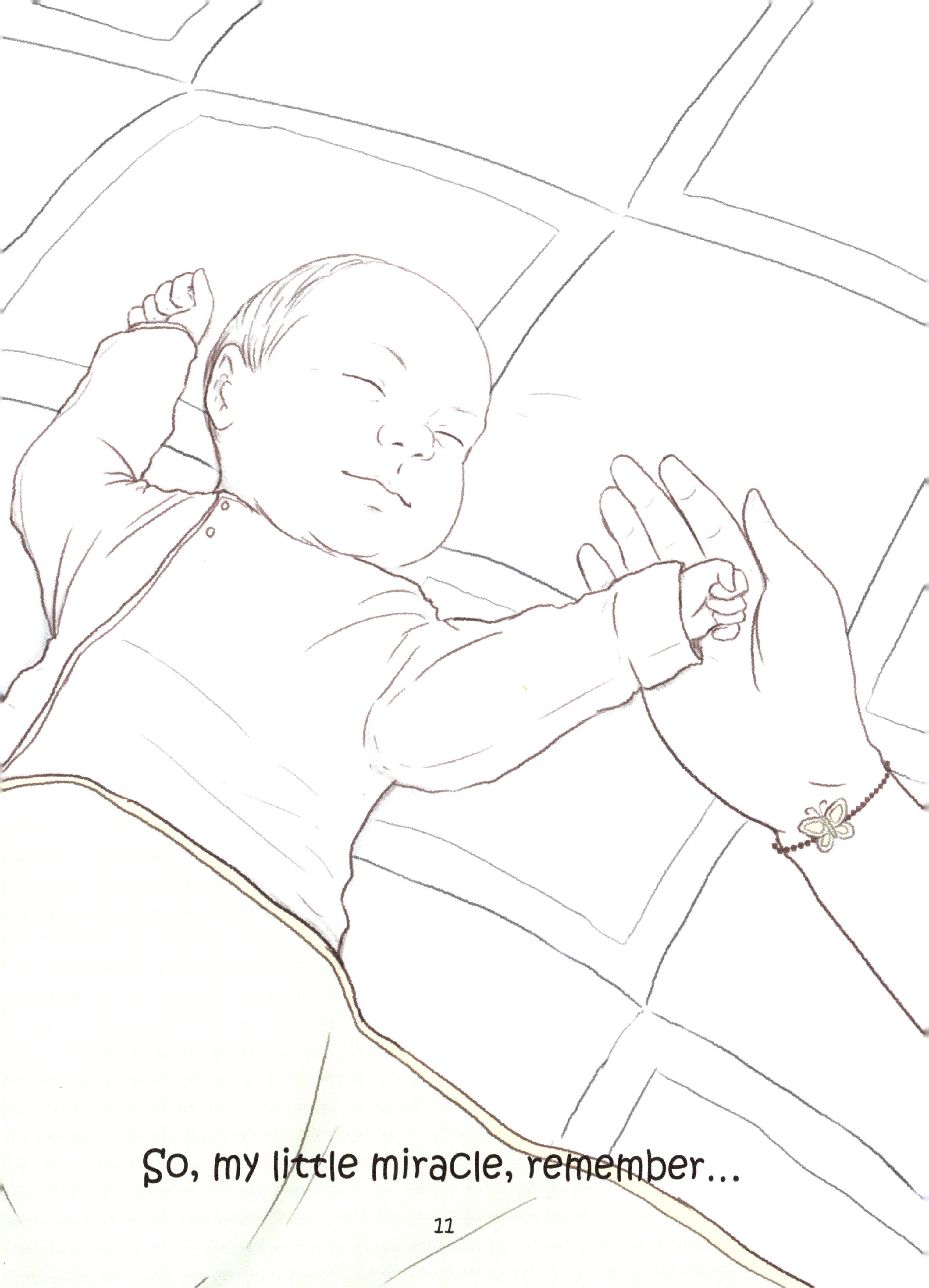

So, my little miracle, remember…

Always seek God first.
Trust His plan for you.

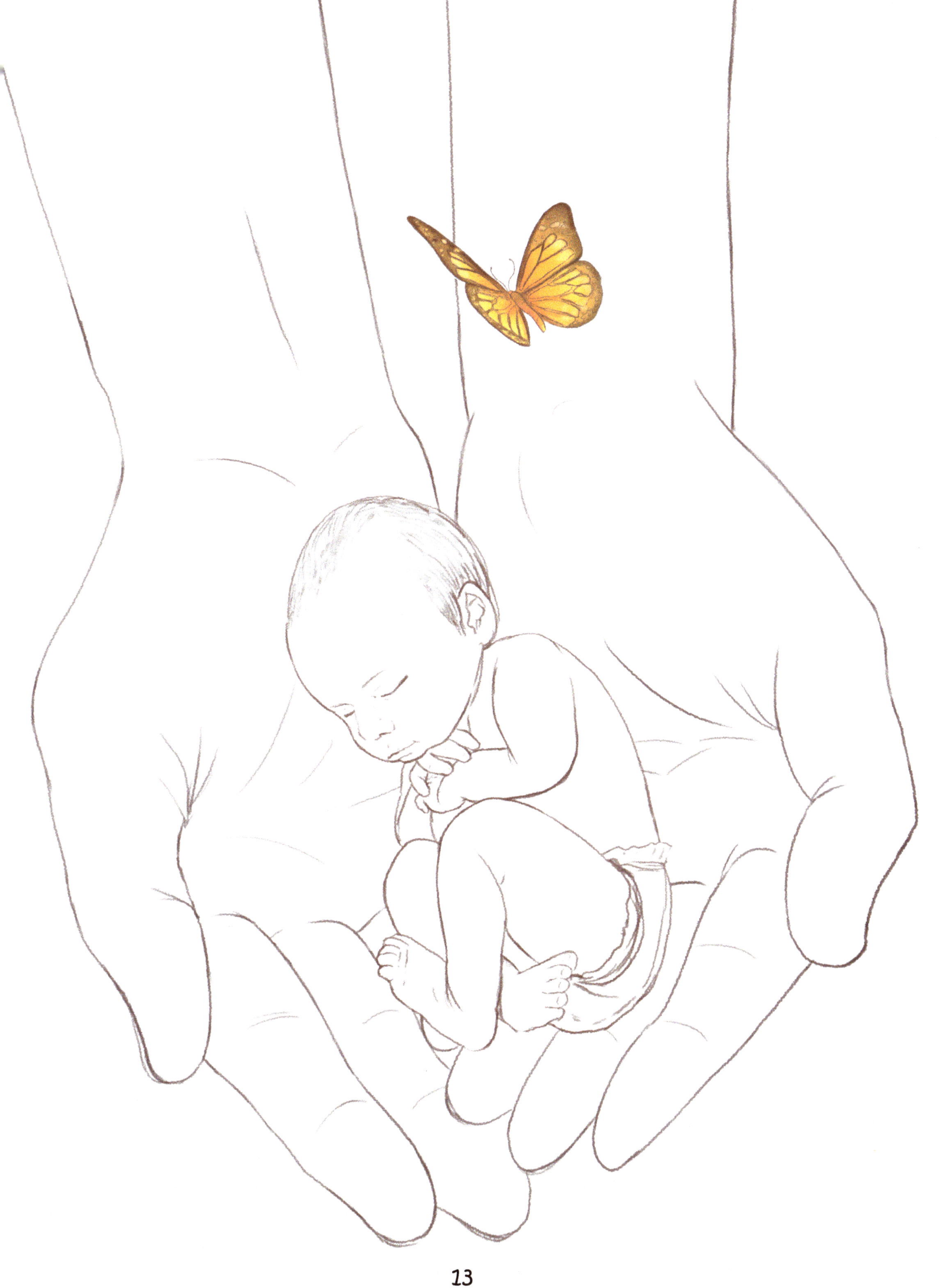

When He speaks…listen.

Listen, and hear Him with an open mind and an open heart.

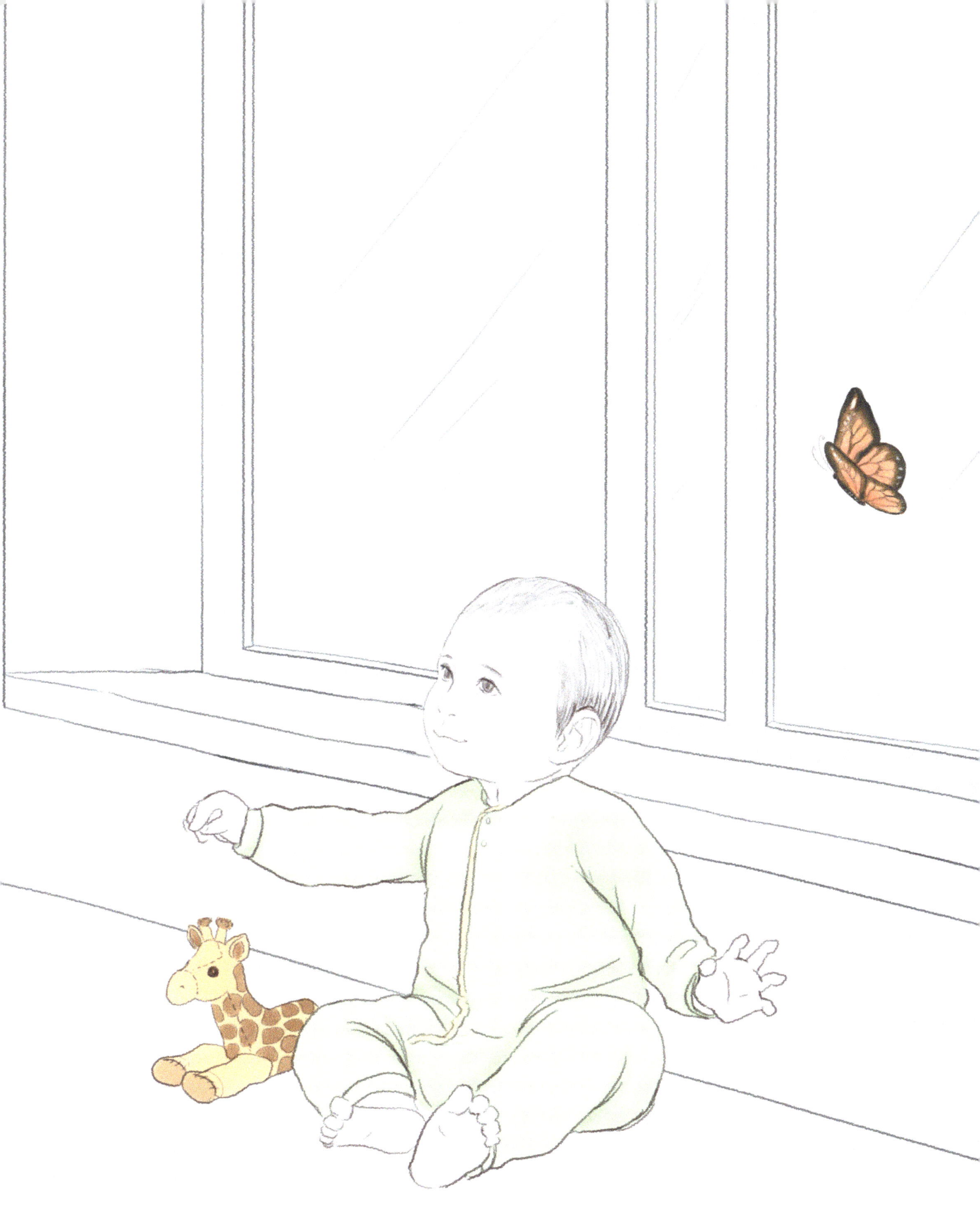

He will light the way for you, for He is
"The Way."

God is always good.

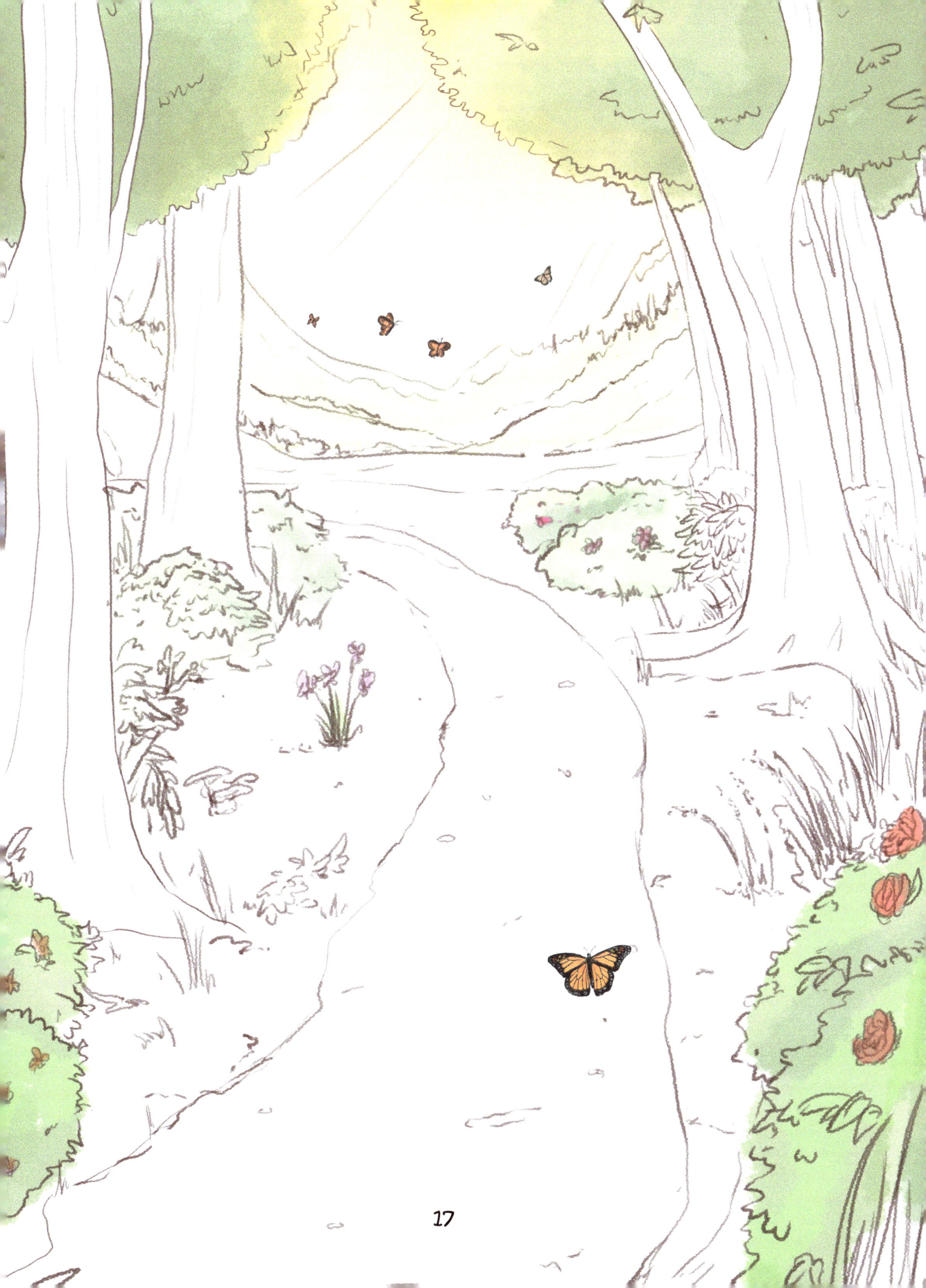

Rejoice in who you are,

a child of God.

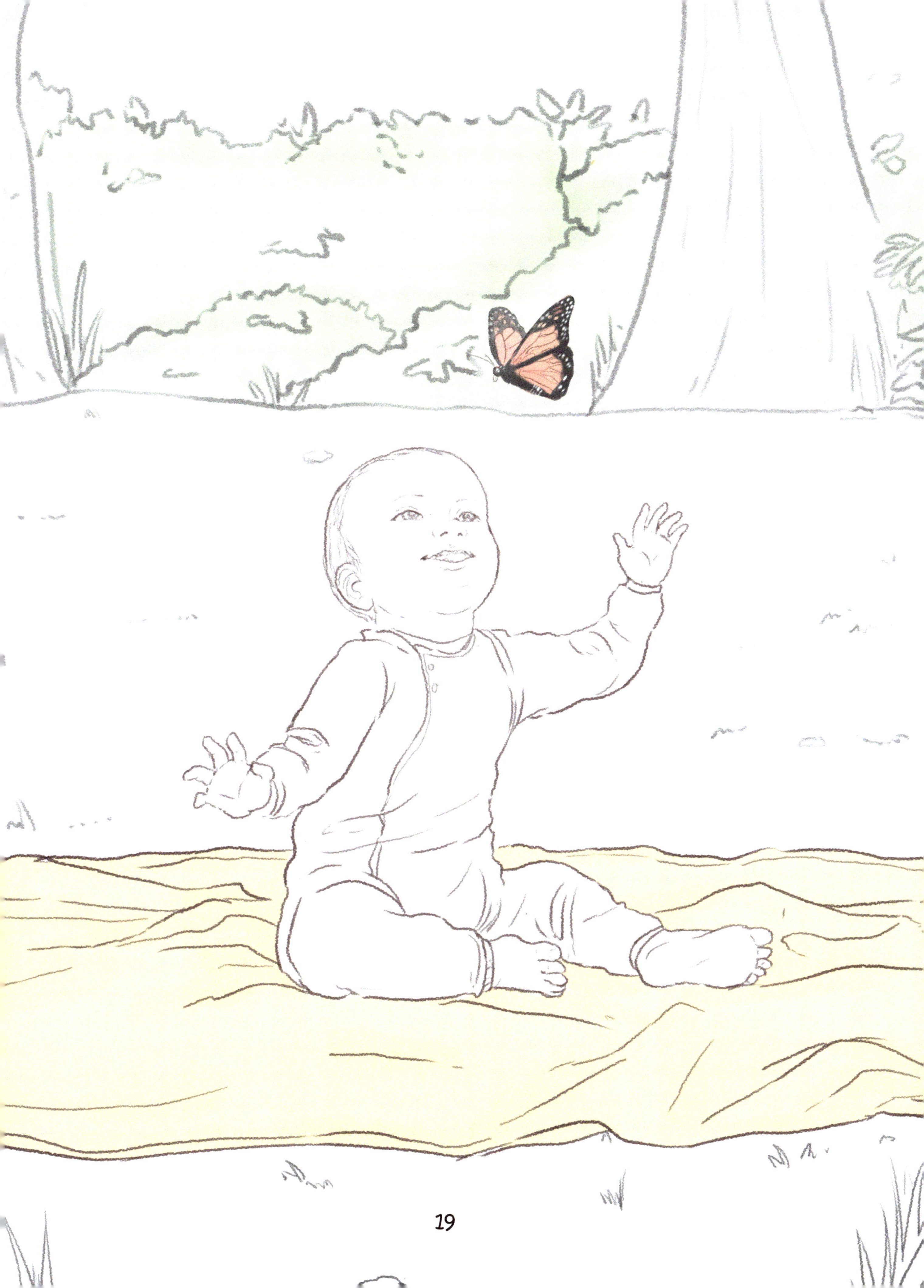

Soon, I will hold you in my arms.

Kiss each of your tiny fingers and toes.

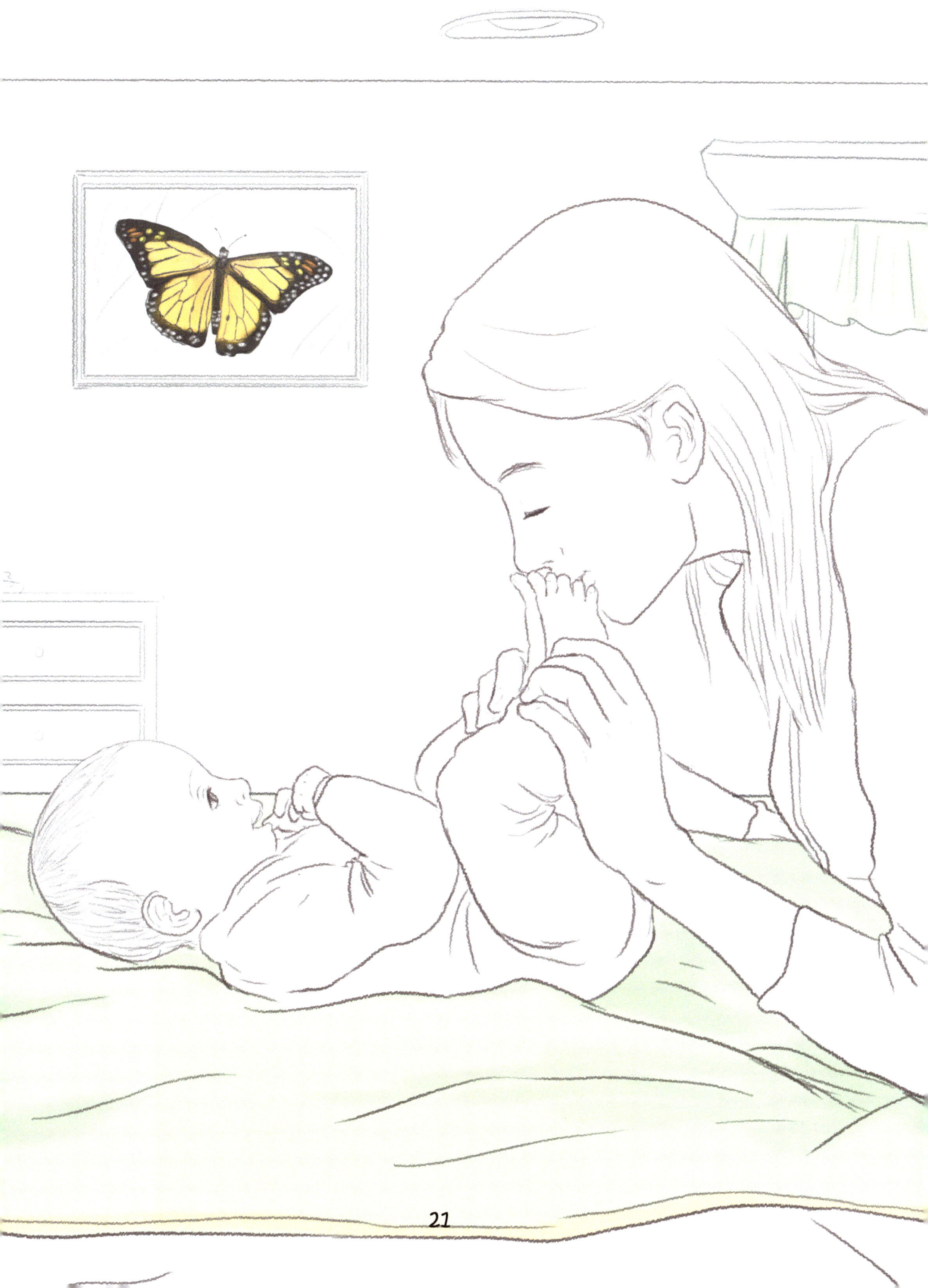

And whisper in your ear,

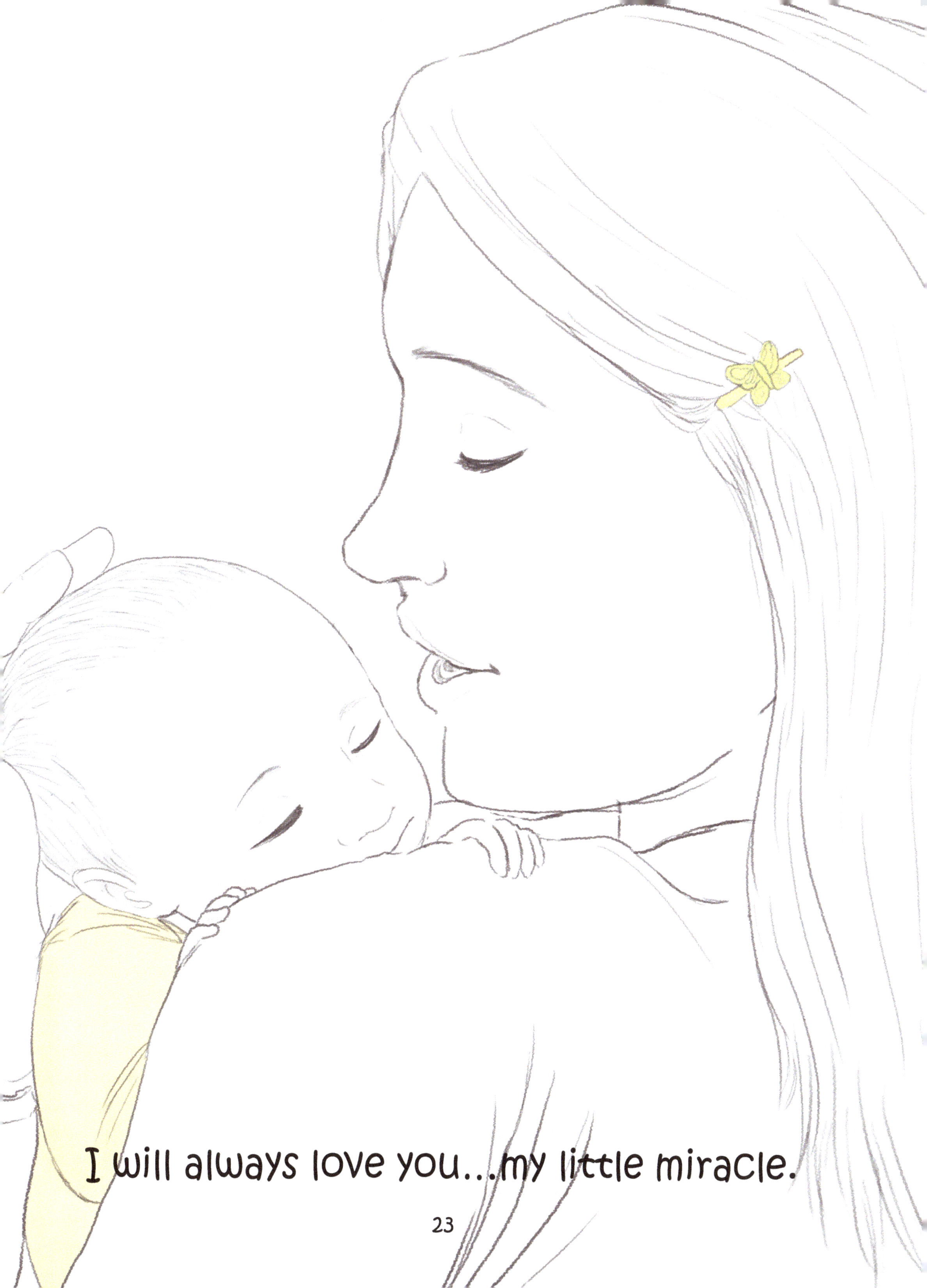

I will always love you...my little miracle.

Corinne Lamontagne earned a bachelor's degree in Elementary Education and a minor in communications from Rhode Island College. She currently teaches third grade and resides with her daughter in Port St. Lucie, Florida. Strong in her faith and a first time author, she credits God as the inspiration for her book.